Digest This Now

...For Kids!

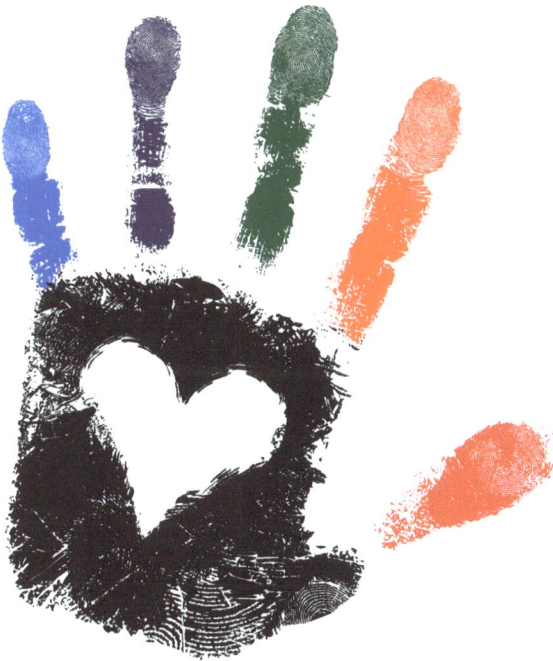

Kai Nunziato-Cruz

Son of Liz Cruz, M.D.
Best Selling Author of *"Answering the Call"* &
Tina Nunziato, Certified Holistic Nutrition Consultant

Digest This Now... For Kids!
By Kai Nunziato-Cruz, Liz Cruz, M.D. & Tina Nunziato, C.H.N.C

Published by www.drlizcruz.com
4110 N. 108th Avenue, Ste. 105
Phoenix, AZ 85037

Cover design by Justin Gonzalez.

This book is not intended to provide medical advice or to take the place of medical advice and treatment from your personal physician. Readers are advised to consult their own doctors or other qualified health professionals regarding the treatment of their medical problems.

Neither the publisher nor the authors take any responsibility for any possible consequences from any treatment, action or application of medicine, supplement, or preparation to any person reading or following the information in this book. If readers are taking prescription medications, they should consult with their physicians and not take themselves off of medicines to start supplementation without the proper supervision of a physician.

This book is dedicated to all the kids in the world that want to be healthy – because without you, there would be no reason for it!

We are so excited to finally deliver this amazing information into your little hands.

We are so grateful to be teaching you at such a young age.

Now let's go out and change the world!

Acknowledgements

We'd like to thank our son Kai Noah Anthony Nunziato-Cruz for taking time out of his busy schedule to spend a long hard weekend with his mommies writing this book. We are so proud of you son!

Thank you to all the little ones that helped us edit this book and make it what it is today. Your input was amazing!

Finally, we would like to thank God for continuing to guide us and remind us how important it is to rely on Him for everything.

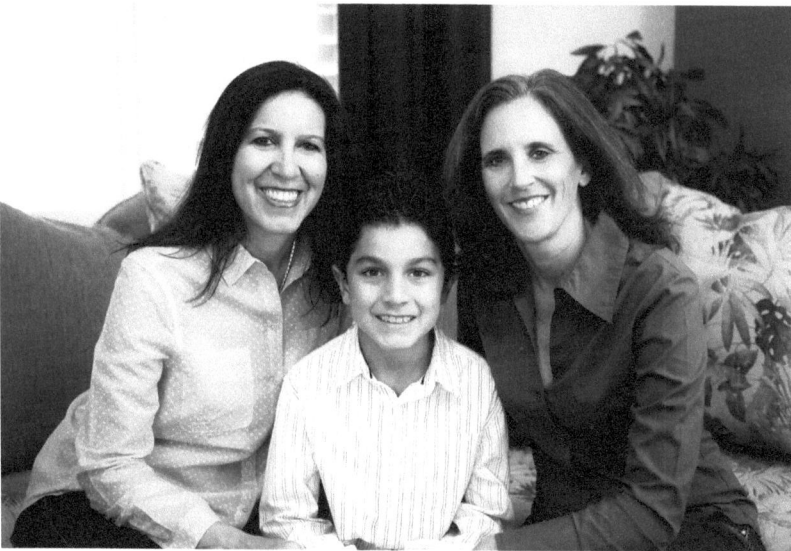

Kai with his Moms when he started his journey in 2013.

Hi, my name is Kai, I am a kid just like you.

My favorite things are playing sports, playing drums and piano, being on stage, riding my skateboard and going to the movies.

I have twin sisters who are younger than me and an older brother.

I am being raised by two Moms who are crazy about eating and drinking healthy and are teaching people about it.

They are helping lots of adults and I feel like it's my turn to help a lot of kids.

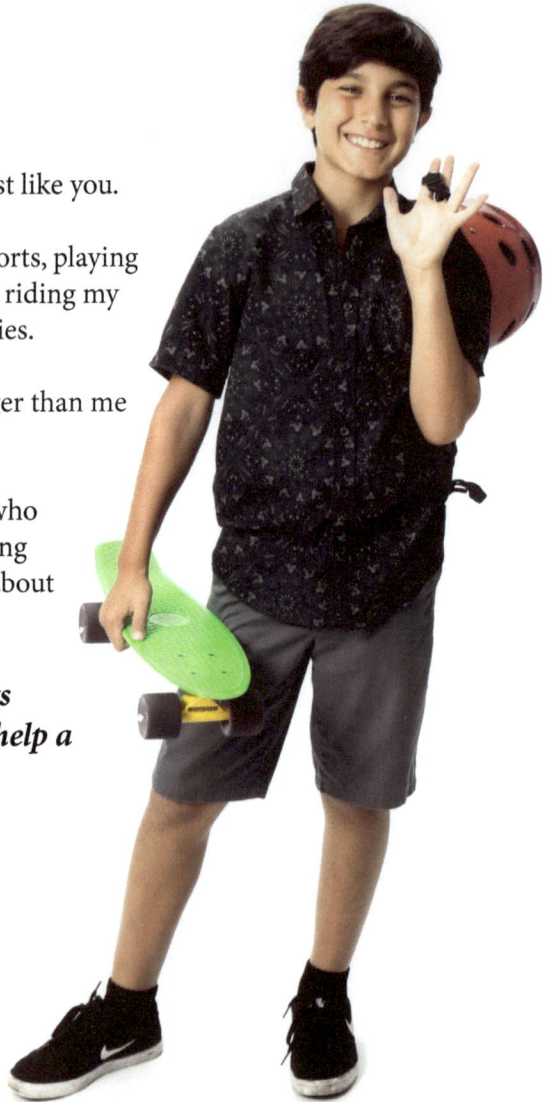

6

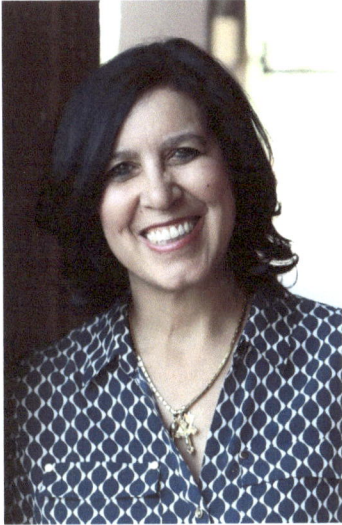

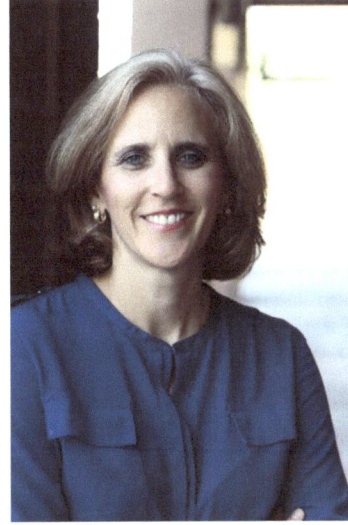

This is my Mom, Dr. Liz Cruz. She is a gastroenterologist which is a big word for doctor of the digestive system, but I like to call her Butt Doctor!

This is my Mom, Tina Nunziato. She is a Certified Holistic Nutritionist which is a long way of saying she teaches you to eat good food and keep your body clean.

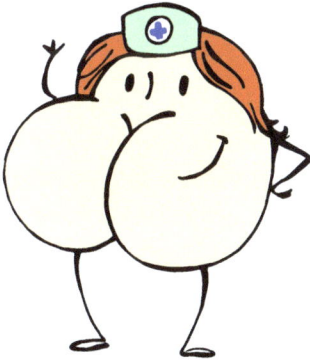

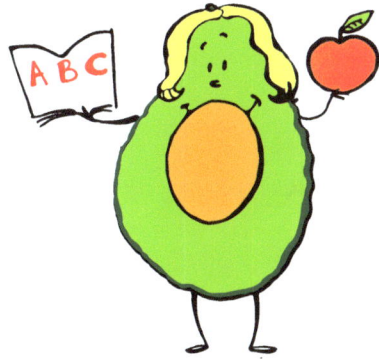

For years, my Moms have been teaching people how to get their body well. They have a medical practice, an online radio show, many books and lots of ways for people to learn. Their love for helping people has rubbed off on me and now I am going to help you!

Here is what I know about kids these days, many of them are...

→ Sick with really bad health problems

→ Having trouble digesting their food

→ Taking lots of medicines

→ Overweight

→ Not getting enough sleep

→ Stressed out

→ Not exercising

→ Eating lots of really bad food and they don't even know it

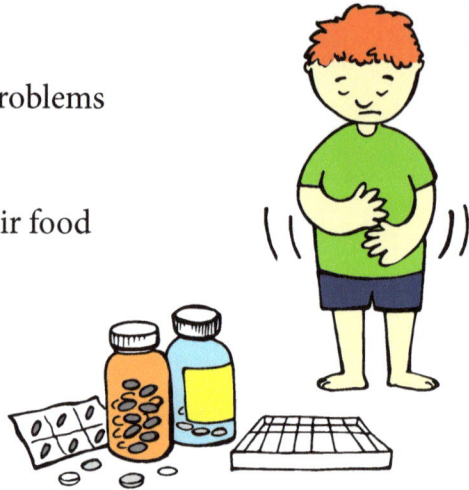

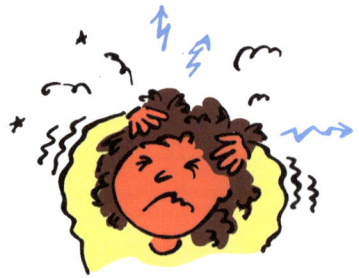

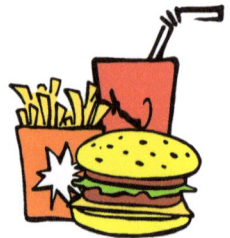

If any of these things describe you, this book is for you!

If you want to get well, it's not hard.

There are some simple things you need to learn and do to get your body healthier and stronger.

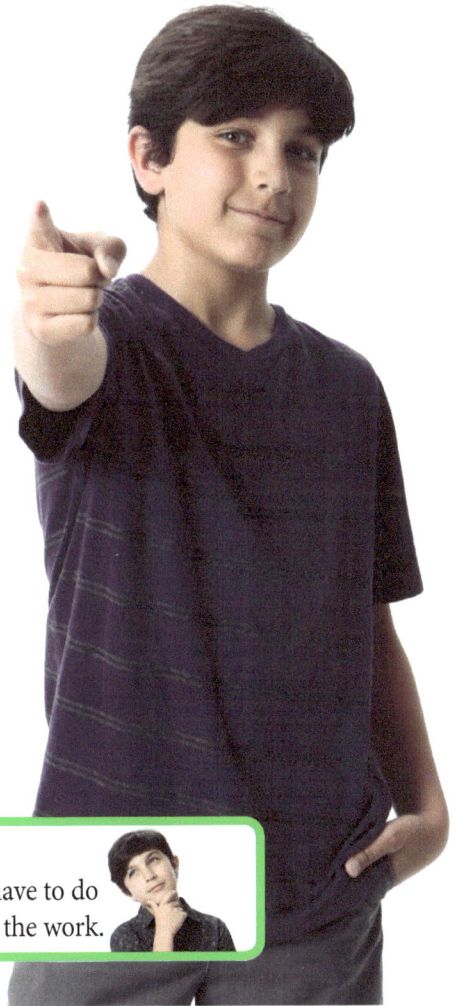

DID YOU KNOW...
Your body can heal itself? All you have to do is give it what it needs and let it do the work.

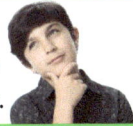

In order to keep your body healthy, you have to learn how it works.

So let's start with the cells in your body.

Your body is made of organs, which are made of tissue, which are made of cells.

You have trillions of cells in your body that each have a special job.

Our body...

Is made up of organs...

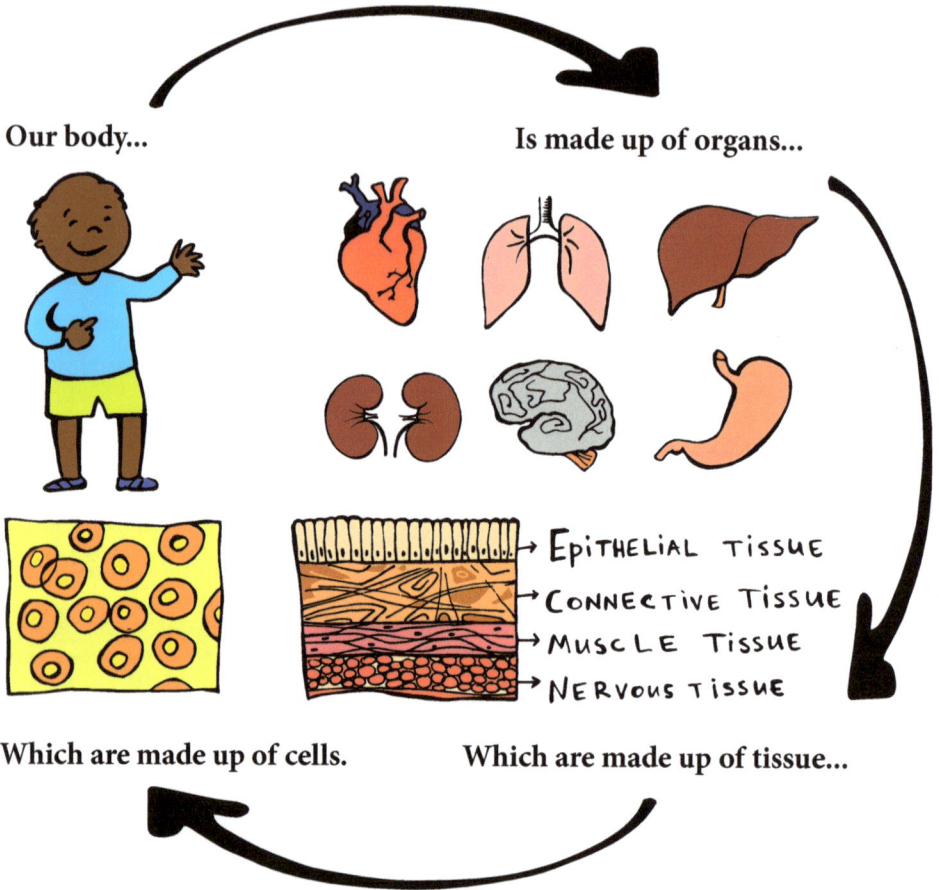

→ EPITHELIAL TISSUE
→ CONNECTIVE TISSUE
→ MUSCLE TISSUE
→ NERVOUS TISSUE

Which are made up of cells.

Which are made up of tissue...

? DID YOU KNOW...
That you have over 37.2 trillion cells in your body?

New cells are being made every day.

If you want to have a healthy body, you must have healthy cells.

The cells in your body need three things to be healthy.

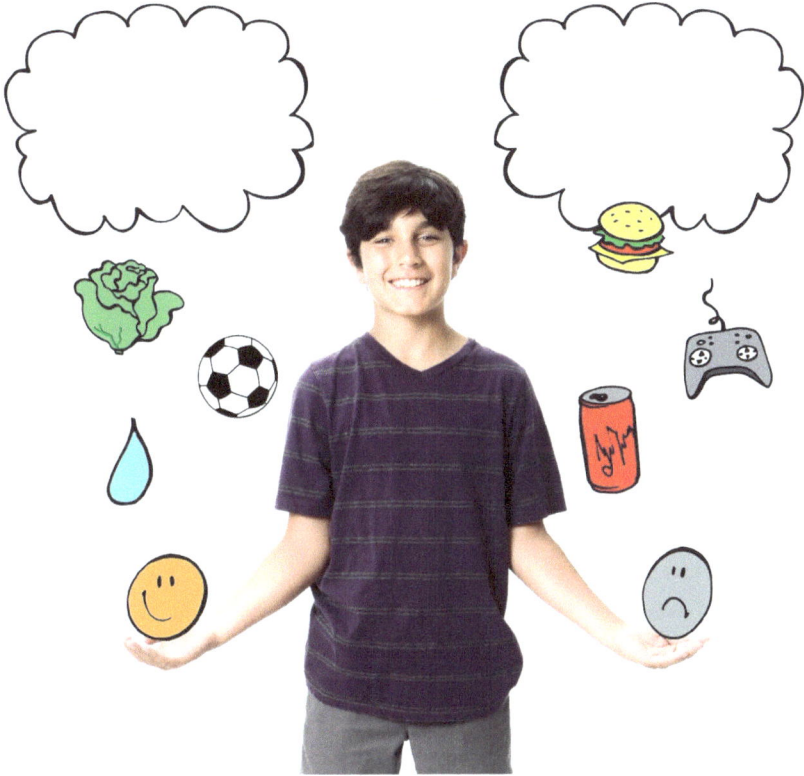

✓ **Good Food** ✓ **Water** ✓ **Oxygen**

Your body is so amazing that your cells can get well quickly just by changing what you are feeding them.

There are certain organs in the body that work really hard to feed you and keep you well.

These include your digestive system and your organs that remove waste from your body.

Let me show you...

Organs of the Digestive System

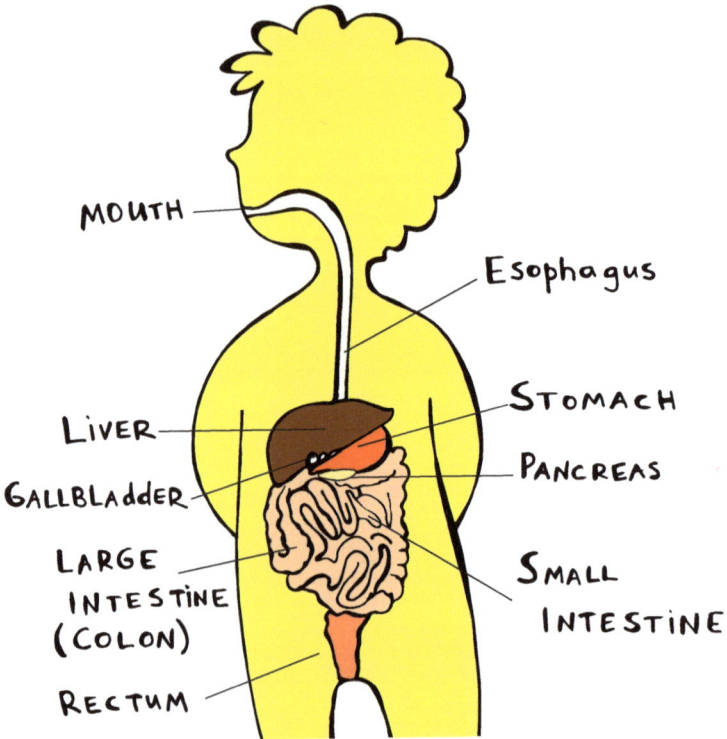

MOUTH

Esophagus

STOMACH

LIVER

PANCREAS

GALLBLADDER

LARGE
INTESTINE
(COLON)

SMALL
INTESTINE

RECTUM

This set of organs is responsible for breaking down and digesting the food you eat and absorbing the nutrients from that food.

It is also responsible for getting rid of stuff the body doesn't need or want... (that's your poop – which comes out at the rectum).

There are other organs that remove unwanted things from your body.

These are called your organs of elimination because they help us eliminate (or get rid of) things our body doesn't want or need.

Organs of Elimination

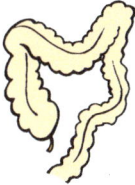

Large Intestine:
Poop / Stool

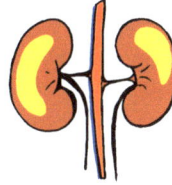

Kidneys:
Pee / Urine

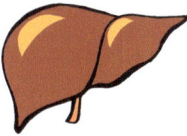

Liver:
Cleaning toxins from the blood

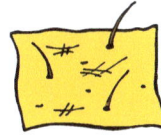

Skin:
Getting rid of toxins through sweat

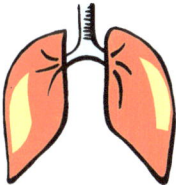

Lungs:
Breathing out toxins

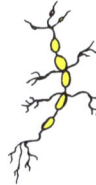

Lymphatic System:
Keeping the body clean from bacteria, viruses and old cells

If your body does not get rid of waste properly it builds up and makes you sick.

DID YOU KNOW...
That every time you eat, you should poop? That means if you eat 3 times per day you should poop 3 times per day. Some people don't even poop one time per day.

This leads into why we are so sick.

There are many reasons this is happening so let me tell you…

☹ We are mostly eating food that is filled with chemicals and sugar.

☹ We are drinking everything but water.

☹ We are not getting rid of waste also known as toxins.

☹ We are stressed out all the time.

☹ We are not getting good rest.

☹ We are not moving our bodies enough.

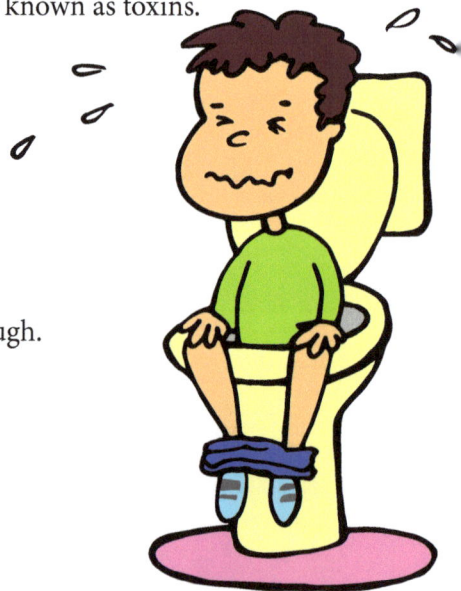

14

And what makes all of this even worse is that doctors are taught to give you medicine for every sickness.

And although medicine does come in handy sometimes, it's not the answer all the time.

Medicines have side effects, which might make you need even more medicine.

My Moms have found that the more medicine someone takes, the sicker their body gets.

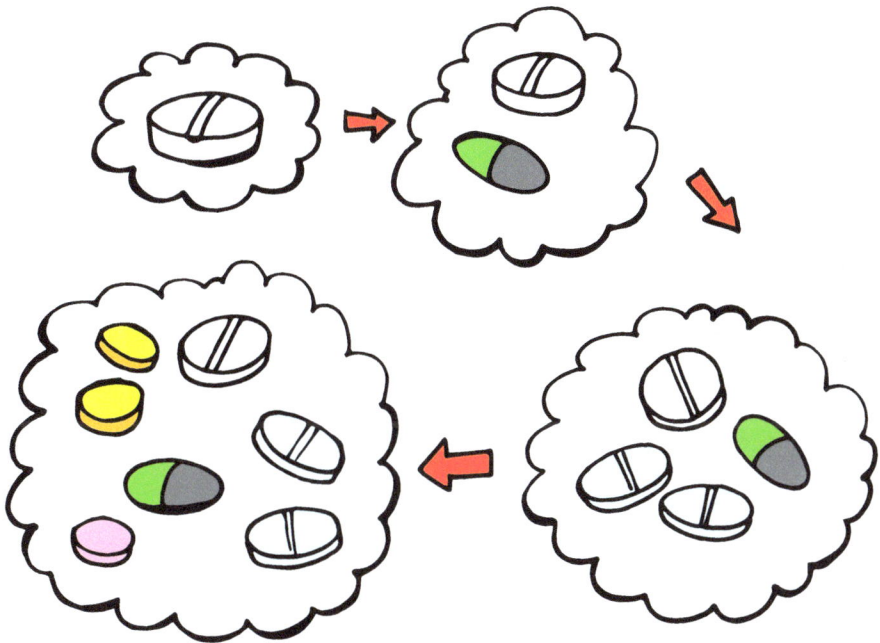

Unfortunately, our medical system is not set up to get us well!

That is why we have to take our health into our own hands.

One of the easiest ways to get healthy is to eat and drink better.

But first let's talk about the food that's making us sick.

Most of the time, we are eating food and drinking beverages that are filled with chemicals and sugar.

Such as:

- Fast foods
- Foods that come from a bag, box, or can that are able to sit on the shelf forever
- Microwaveable foods
- Candy, cakes, cookies, donuts, ice cream
- Animal meat (chickens, cows, and pigs) or food that comes from animals (milk, cheese, and eggs) which have all been pumped with hormones and antibiotics
- Sodas, energy drinks, sports drinks, fancy coffees, and juices

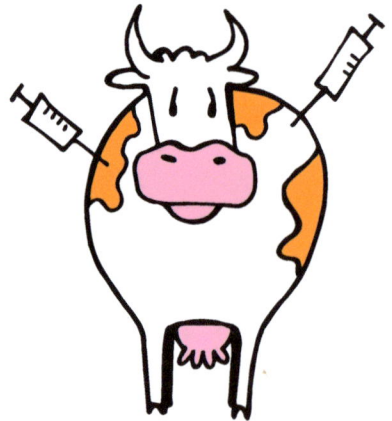

These items are loaded with chemicals and sugar and have very few healthy nutrients.

The chemicals and sugar are like poison to your body.

DID YOU KNOW...
That most yogurts have a ton of sugar and chemicals in them? And here you thought they were healthy.

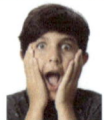

So why do we eat like this?

Over the last 30 to 40 years the people in our country have asked for fast and cheap food and that's exactly what we got.

We never thought about how this fast, cheap food would affect our health.

Still to this day, most people do not understand how food and drink affects their body.

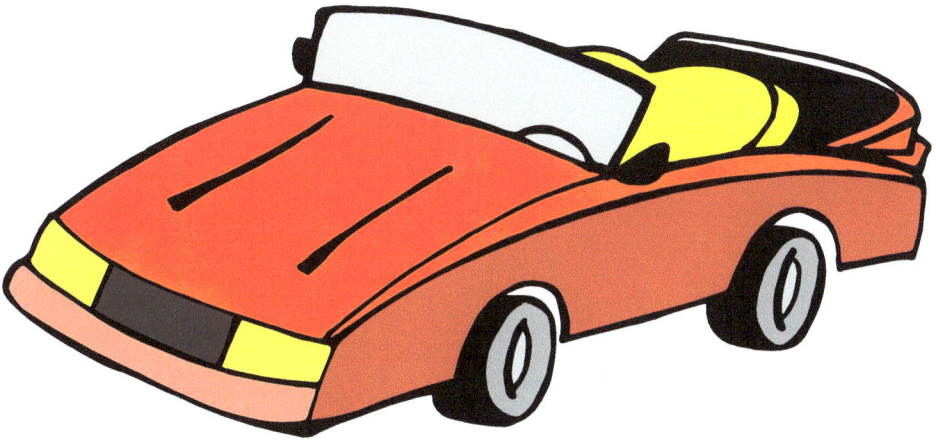

Think of your body like a car.

In order for a car to work well you have to give it gas, oil changes and regular repairs and maintenance.

If you don't, your car will break down.

This is the same thing that happens to your body.

You have to give it gas (good food, water and oxygen), oil changes (going to the bathroom and sweating) and regular repairs and maintenance (movement and good sleep).

Speaking of good sleep, why is sleep so important for your body?

It's during sleep that your body and your cells, rest, repair and recharge.

Think of your body as a cell phone.

During the day while the phone is being used the battery runs out.

In order to keep using the phone it has to recharge for a period of time.

The same goes for your body.

In order to stay healthy and have energy, you must spend time every night recharging.

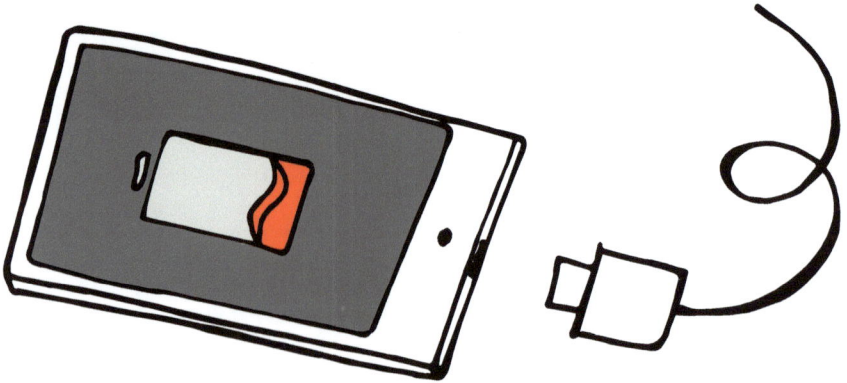

DID YOU KNOW...
That your body is hard at work while you are sleeping? Every night your liver processes all the blood in your body and cleans it. If you are not in bed sleeping during this process your liver cannot do its job properly.

Kids Are Stressed Too…

Being stressed out all the time can also make your body sick.

It's common for adults to be stressed but I have friends my age that are stressed out all the time.

They stress about their home life, school, after school activities, friendships, and being pressured by friends to do things.

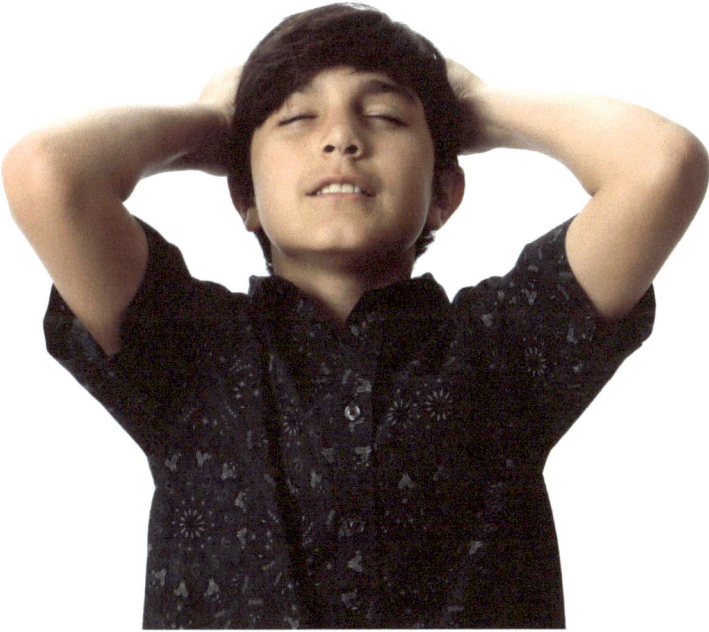

We are so worried about the pressures we feel on the outside, we don't realize the pressure stress puts on the inside of our body.

Now let's talk about movement.

As I'm sure you know most kids these days are spending lots of time watching TV, being on the computer, playing video games and playing on our tablets and cell phones.

These types of activities have replaced being active outside and playing in sports, what my Moms like to call moving your body.

Not only are we not building up strong muscles by not moving we can't get rid of the waste (toxins) easily.

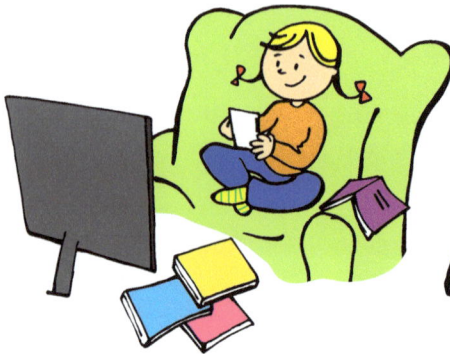

Energy / Life Level   Energy / Life Level

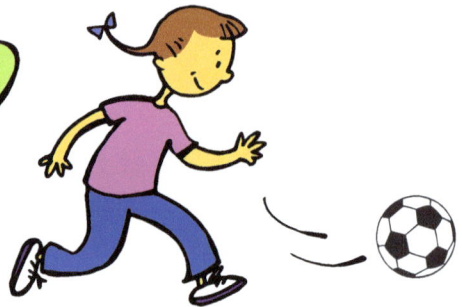

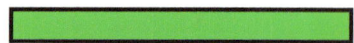

DID YOU KNOW...
That your lymph system (a system in your body that helps to clean out toxins) only moves when you move. If this system gets backed up you can get sick.

Wow!

That was a lot of information.

Now you know why there are so many sick and overweight adults and kids in the United States.

And if they are not sick and overweight now, they probably will be soon if they continue living this way.

There was a study done by the American Medical Association in 2012 that said we are the first generation of kids that may not live past our parents.

I don't know about you but this makes me so sad and mad at the same time.

This is not right and must be changed…are you with me?

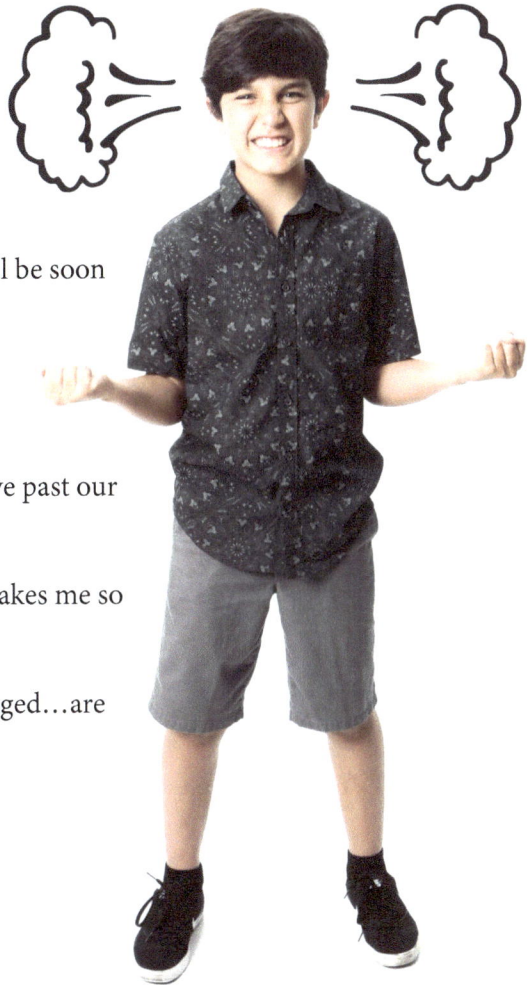

I want you to know we as a generation can change the world.

We are the future!

We can decide that we don't want to be sick and overweight any more.

We don't want to be on medicines any more.

We don't want our parents or family members getting sick any more.

Let's spend the rest of the book talking about how we are going to get the world well!

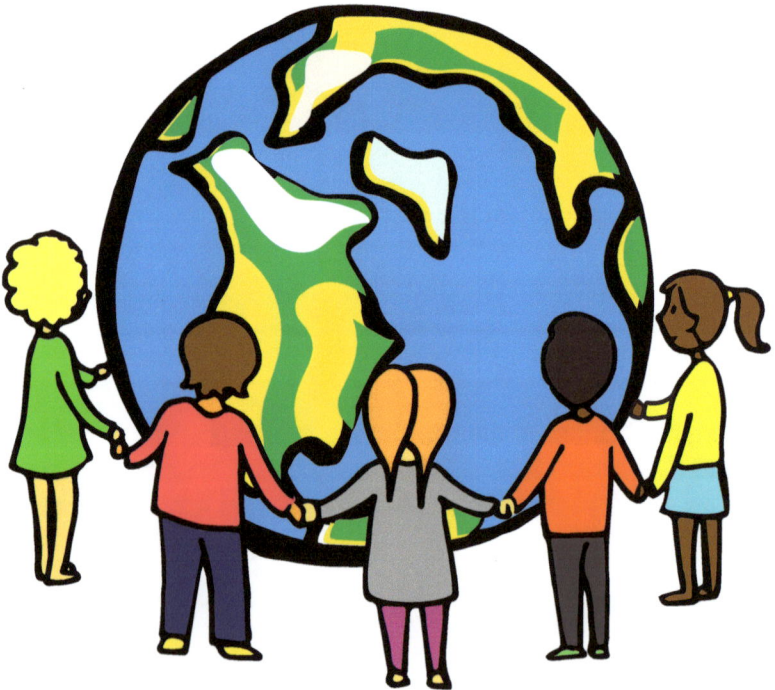

To begin, here's what you need to learn…

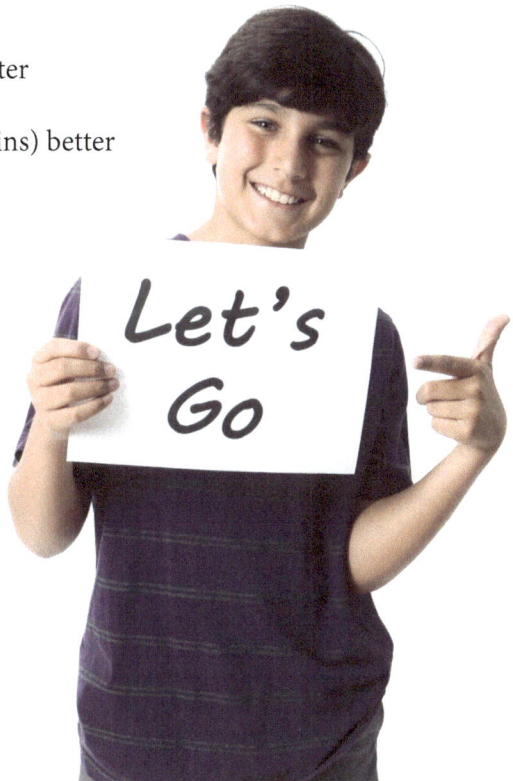

☺ Healthy foods to eat

☺ Healthy drinks to drink

☺ How to digest your food better

☺ How to get rid of waste (toxins) better

☺ How to get better rest

☺ How to stress less

☺ How to move more

☺ How to join a generation that's changing the world

The best way to teach you about healthy food is by breaking down the bad and the good by the food groups.

On this page you will see a list of not so good foods and on the next page you will see a list of much healthier foods.

The Dirty List

Proteins: Chicken, Turkey, Beef (burgers, hot dogs, steak, ribs), Pork (bacon, sausage, ham), Lunch Meat, Farm Raised Fish, Peanut Butter, Eggs

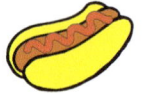

Carbs / Grains: White Rice, White / Wheat Pasta, White / Wheat Bread (Pizza) and Biscuits, Crackers, Chips, Flour Tortillas, Oatmeal, Waffles, Pancakes, Bagels, Muffins, Boxed Cereals

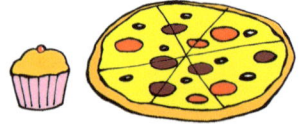

Vegetables: Iceberg Lettuce, White / Red Potatoes, Corn, Mushrooms, Canned or Frozen Vegetables

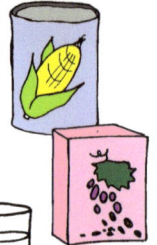

Fruits: Dried, Pickled or Canned Fruit, Processed Fruit Snacks, Fruit Cups

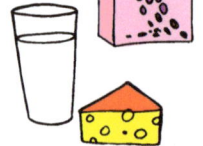

Dairy: Cow's Milk, Cheese, Yogurt, Creamers, Sour Cream, Cream Cheese, Ice Cream

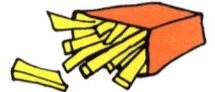

Fats: Vegetable Oil, Canola Oil, Butter from Cow's Milk, Salad Dressings, French Fries, Fried Foods

Sugars: Cakes, Donuts, Cookies, Chocolates, Candy, Syrups, Jelly, Artificial Sugars (Aspartame, Sweet-n-low, Equal, Splenda)

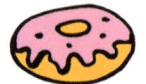

You might be thinking what's left to eat, I'll tell you what's left to eat – REAL FOOD!

And it tastes so good! I dare you to give it a try!

The Clean List

Proteins: Chicken, Beef and Pork that are all grass fed, hormone and antibiotic free, Wild Caught Fish (salmon, mahi, cod, orange roughy, sea bass, tuna, shrimp), Veggie Burgers, Soy Patties, Tofu, Tempeh, Hummus, Beans (kidney, black, garbanzo, lentils, pinto, red, soy, navy, great northern), Nut / Seed Butters (almond, cashew, hazelnut, sunflower), Quinoa, Hemp Seeds, Chia Seeds, Green Vegetables (you get lots of proteins by eating greens)

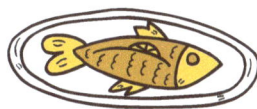

Carbs / Grains: Brown Rice, Wild Rice, Jasmine Rice, Quinoa, Millet, Spelt, Brown Rice Pasta, Quinoa Pasta, Rice Noodles, Buckwheat Noodles, Ezekiel Bread, Corn Tortillas, Buckwheat Pancakes

Vegetables: Lettuces (Red Leaf, Green Leaf, Romaine, Spinach, Arugula, Kale, Mixed Greens), Sweet Potatoes, Yams, Purple Potatoes, Fresh Vegetables such as Artichokes, Asparagus, Beets, Bell Peppers, Bok Choy, Broccoflower / Broccoli, Brussels Sprouts, Cabbage, Carrots, Cauliflower, Celery, Collard / Mustard Greens, Cucumber, Endive, Escarole, Garlic, Green Beans, Leeks, Okra, Radish, Rhubarb, Rutabaga, Spinach, Sprouts, Swiss Chard, Tomato, Turnip, Zucchini

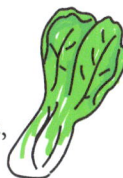

Fruits: Any Fresh Fruit – but don't eat too much if you are trying to lose weight

Dairy: Almond Milk, Soy Milk, Rice Milk, Hemp Milk, Coconut Milk and consider buying cheese, butter and ice cream made from these milks

Fats: Olive Oil, Avocado Oil, Flaxseed Oil, Grape Seed Oil, Hemp Oil, Sunflower Oil (oils should always be eaten raw never cooked), Avocados, Fish, Raw Nuts and Seeds (walnuts, almonds, pecans, pumpkin seeds, sunflower seeds)

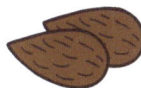

Sugars: Stevia, Raw Honey, Grade B Maple Syrup, Coconut Palm Sugar, Coconut Nectar, Agave Nectar, at our house we use fresh fruit as our form of sugar.

This is our version of a healthy food pyramid.

Here's how it works… at the bottom is what you want to be eating all the time and at the top is what you want to be eating the least.

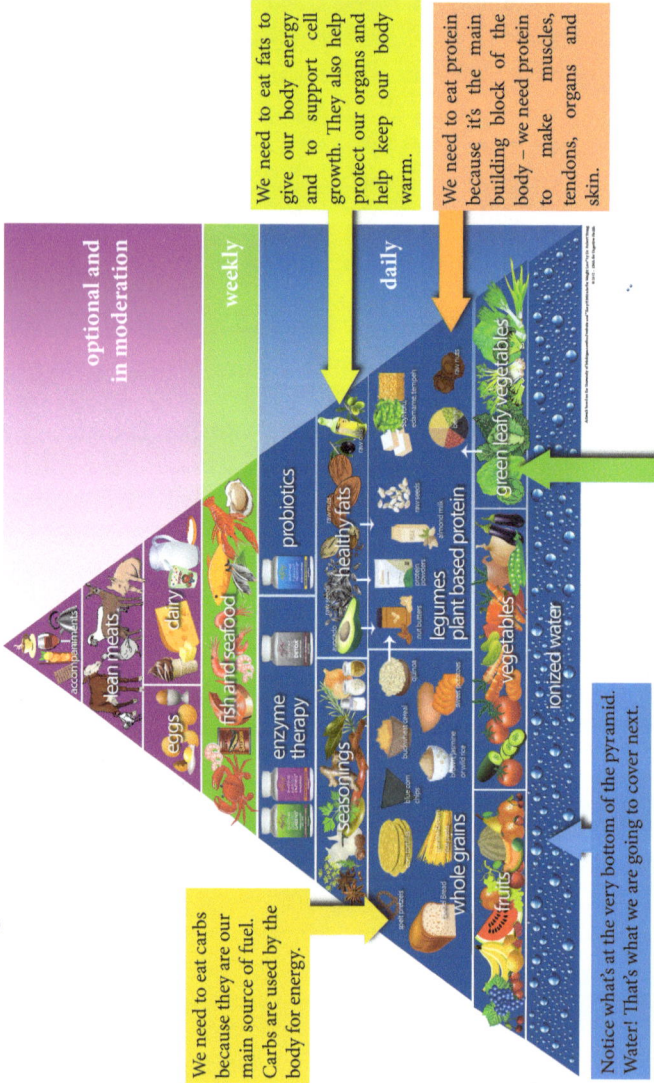

We need to eat fats to give our body energy and to support cell growth. They also help protect our organs and help keep our body warm.

We need to eat protein because it's the main building block of the body – we need protein to make muscles, tendons, organs and skin.

optional and in moderation

weekly

daily

supplements

lean meats

eggs

dairy

fish and seafood

enzyme therapy

seasonings

probiotics

healthy fats

legumes plant based protein

green leafy vegetables

vegetables

whole grains

fruits

ionized water

We need to eat carbs because they are our main source of fuel. Carbs are used by the body for energy.

Notice what's at the very bottom of the pyramid. Water! That's what we are going to cover next.

Greens have more nutrition per calorie than any other food – they are packed with all the vitamins and minerals that the body needs to work properly. If you don't like eating greens you absolutely must consider supplementing them. Our Gastro Greens™ are a great source of real plant based vitamins and minerals.

Why do you think water was at the bottom of the food pyramid?

Your body is about 80% water.

You have water in your blood, bones, cells, eyes, brain, you get the idea.

In fact, we are 80% SALT water.

If you have ever tasted your sweat or your tears, you know they are salty.

Every day you lose salt water, when you sweat, when you talk and when you urinate.

In order to have a healthy body you must replace the salt water you are losing each day.

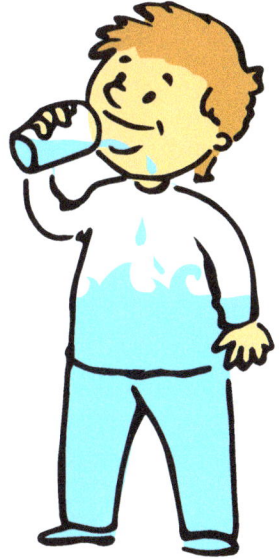

However, we seem to hydrate with everything but water (especially sugary and caffeinated drinks) like the following:

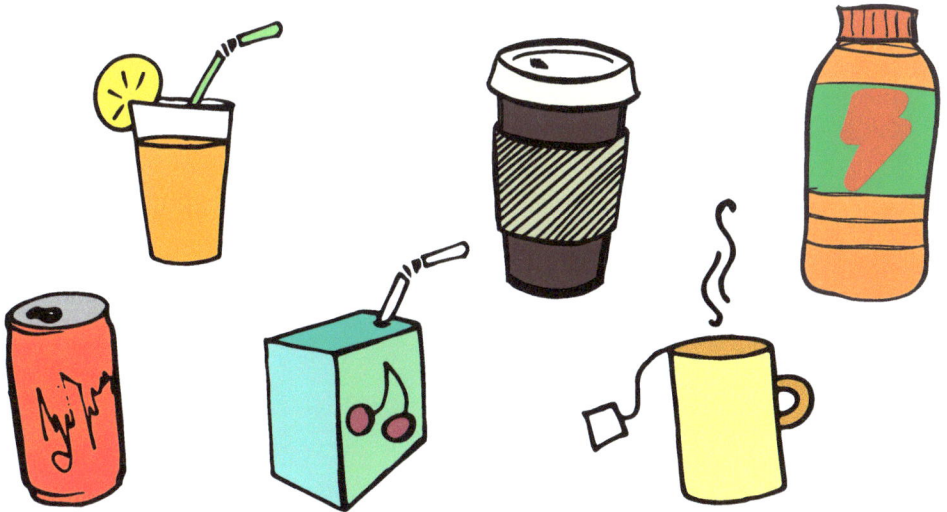

The only thing that hydrates the body is water.

And if you want to get salty water you must drink your electrolytes.

Electrolytes are absolutely necessary in your body for sending messages between your cells so they can work with each other properly.

Electrolytes can be found in sports drinks like Gatorade and Powerade; however, those drinks also have a lot of sugar in them.

We already know that sugar is like poison in the body.

So instead of sports drinks try putting Super Salts™ in your water.

Here is how you can hydrate your body properly…

1. Find out how much you weigh.
2. Divide that number in half.
3. That's the amount of water in ounces you should be drinking each day.
4. For every 12oz of water you drink you should be adding ½ teaspoon of Super Salts™.

Let me show you my numbers…

I weigh 80 pounds. Divide that in half and you have 40 pounds. That means I should be drinking 40 ounces of water per day. I have a 26 ounce water bottle I use every day, which means I should be drinking about 2 water bottles each day with 1 teaspoon of salts in each water bottle.

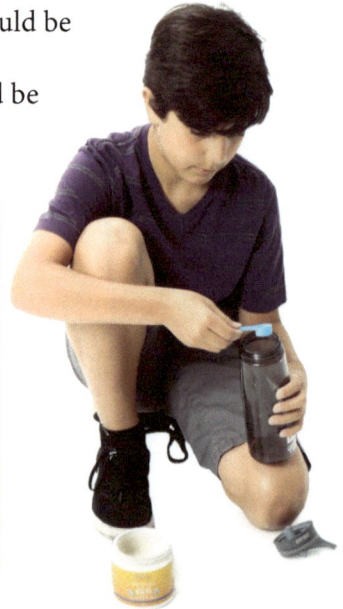

The best way to get your body healthy is to eat real "whole" foods and drink more water, but some kids have lots of problems digesting their food, even if they are eating and drinking healthier.

Things kids may experience are constipation (where you don't poop every day), stomachaches, gas, bloating, regurgitation, reflux, nausea and vomiting.

If you are experiencing any of these issues you should consider taking enzymes and probiotics.

Here is a little lesson on digesting food…

When you eat, food goes into your stomach as a solid.

Your body, cannot use food in a solid form, it has to be broken down into a liquid.

That means when you eat, your body has to go to work.

It has to make enzymes and acid to break your food down properly.

Once the food is liquefied it moves into the small intestine and that is where it gets absorbed into the body.

That is how we feed our body and cells.

When you are not eating a good nutritious diet, it is hard for your body to make the enzymes it needs.

So when you eat, the acid is getting made but not the enzymes.

In order to fix this problem you can start by eating healthy to see if that solves the problem.

If not try taking digestive enzymes every time you eat.

The enzymes will help to break down your food, so it can move on properly in hopes of relieving the digestive issues.

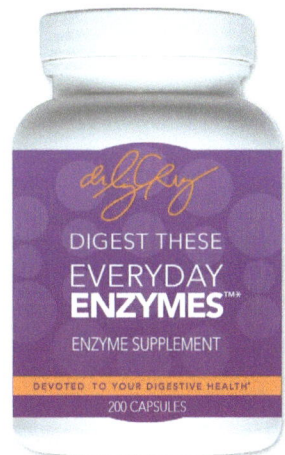

Another great thing to consider are probiotics.

Probiotics are good healthy bacteria (bugs).

You have trillions of bacteria (bugs) living in your intestine.

One of the roles of the bacteria is to keep the gut healthy.

Your gut plays a very important role in keeping the body healthy.
In fact, about 80% of your immune system is in your gut.

We are supposed to have more good bacteria in our gut than bad bacteria.

This balance of bacteria can get thrown off by the food we eat, stress, taking antibiotics and other medicines.

If there is too much bad bacteria and not enough good bacteria you can have symptoms such as gas, bloating, diarrhea, constipation, and stomach pain.

By taking a healthy probiotic every day and flooding your gut with good healthy bacteria (bugs), you can reset the gut and eliminate the symptoms.

DID YOU KNOW...
That all of our capsules can be taken apart and the powder can be put on food or in water. This makes it really easy for kids of all ages to benefit from them.

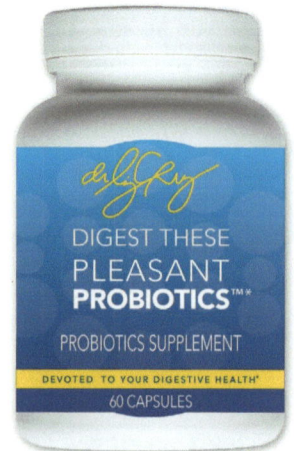

Now let's dive into getting rid of all that waste (toxins) that have built up in the body.

There are some pretty simple things you can do to clean out your body.

1. Drink lots of water

2. Eat lots of soup

3. Drink lots of smoothies

4. If you're not pooping, consider taking our

   Everyday Enzymes™ and Pleasant Probiotics™

5. Move to the point of sweating

6. Consider taking our Delicate Detox™

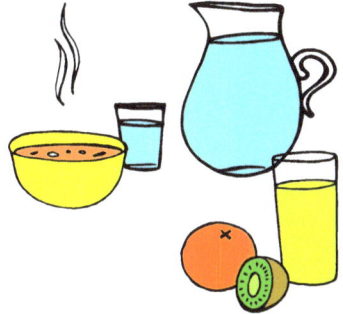

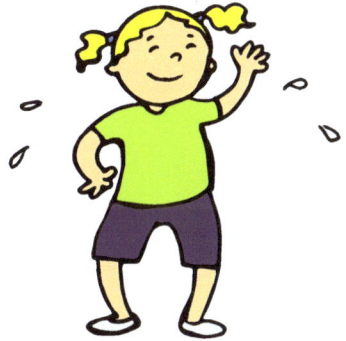

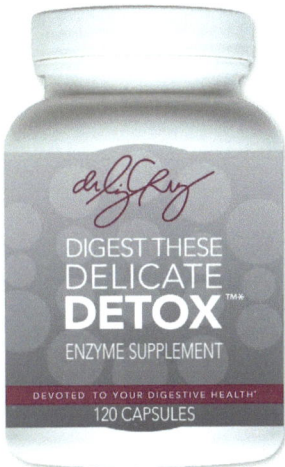

The Delicate Detox™ is a safe and gentle way to clean up the waste (toxins) in your blood.

Next up – stress.

Unfortunately I can't teach you how to take away your stress.

Stress is a natural part of life.

How about I show you some really groovy ways to manage your stress.

With two younger sisters I have had to use these techniques many times.

1. **Get away to a quiet place** and just sit and relax your body and mind.
2. **Practice deep breathing** – take a deep breath in, hold it for 10 seconds and then slowly release it. Do this for at least a minute or two at a time.
3. **Try not to think about or worry about things** that haven't happened yet. One of my favorite quotes is by Mark Twain – *"I've had a lot of worries in my life, most of which never happened."*
4. **Journaling** is a great way to release your stress and anxiety – get the stuff out of your head and put it on paper.
5. **Take time to pray** – whether you believe in God or some other higher being, just know that no matter what you are going through, everything will be okay. Have hope that you can get through anything.

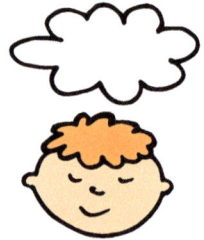

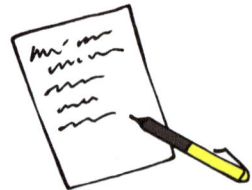

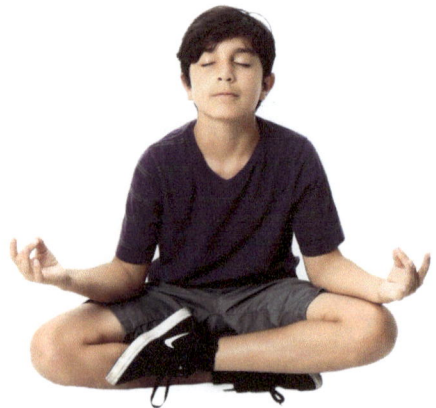

It's time to talk about the most important 8 hours of your day.

Depending on your age you may need a little more, but we all need rest and as kids we should be getting at least 8 hours per night.

Here are some simple tips for making those 8 hours count.

- Try to be in bed before 9pm.

- Sleep in a room that is quiet and dark.

- Try to keep your bed a place for sleeping only – don't watch TV or play games in bed.

- Avoid being in front of a screen at least 30 minutes before bed.

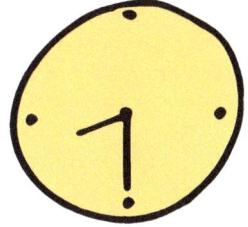

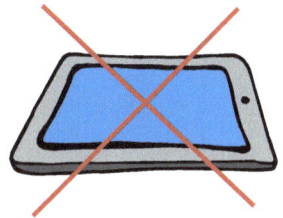

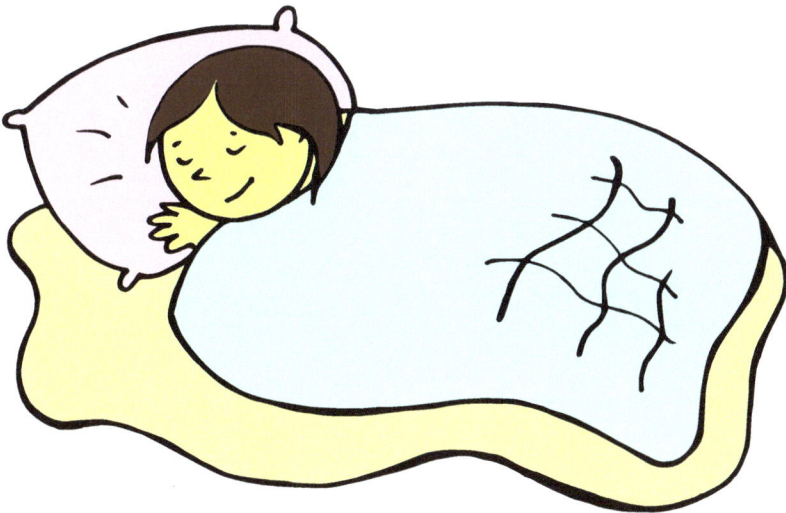

The final lesson, how to move your body.

If you are an active kid and move your body now, I encourage you to keep it up.

Do whatever you can to spend more time being active then sitting in front of a screen.

If you haven't moved your body in a while there are some simple things you can do to get going.

1. Tell your parents to hide your tablet, phone, TV remotes, video game controllers, etc.

2. Spend time looking for them – this gets you moving.

3. When you give up, go outside and play.

Just kidding!

But you should at least consider setting time limits for yourself in front of your favorite screens, for example 30 minutes per day.

Have a plan for yourself on what you will do with the rest of your time.

Like go outside and play, join a sport, ride your bike, go to the skate park, walk your dog, etc.

Your goal should be to move your body for at least 30 minutes every day.

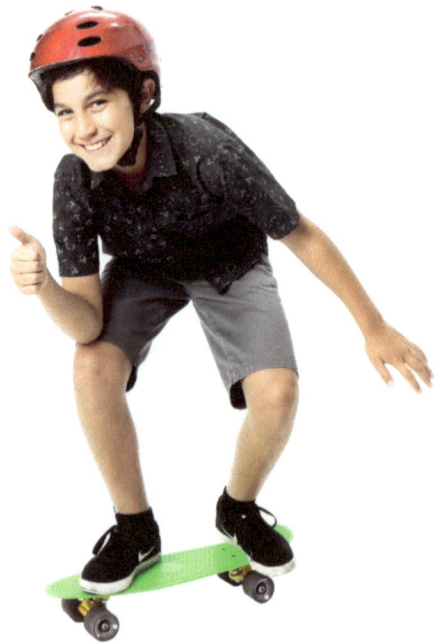

I hope you learned a lot from this book.

I know it's a lot to "digest" get it?

But it's information that can change your life for the better.

Read the book over and over and use it as a daily resource.

If you have a lot of changes to make, make them slowly.

Pick one or two things you can work on and then slowly add things to constantly improve your health and your body.

It took my Moms two years to switch what we were eating.

There is no hurry, just know you are moving toward a goal.

Use the space below to right down your top 5 goals for getting healthier:

1. ---
   ----

2. ---
   ----

3. ---
   ----

4. ---
   ----

5. ---

Every day you have to make an effort to make healthy choices.

It's an ongoing journey.

If you feel like you need more support and guidance I would love for you to join me at:

generationkai.com

For a simple monthly membership you can get plugged in and learn how to change the world!

And don't forget to subscribe to my YouTube channel too!

generationkai.com/youtube

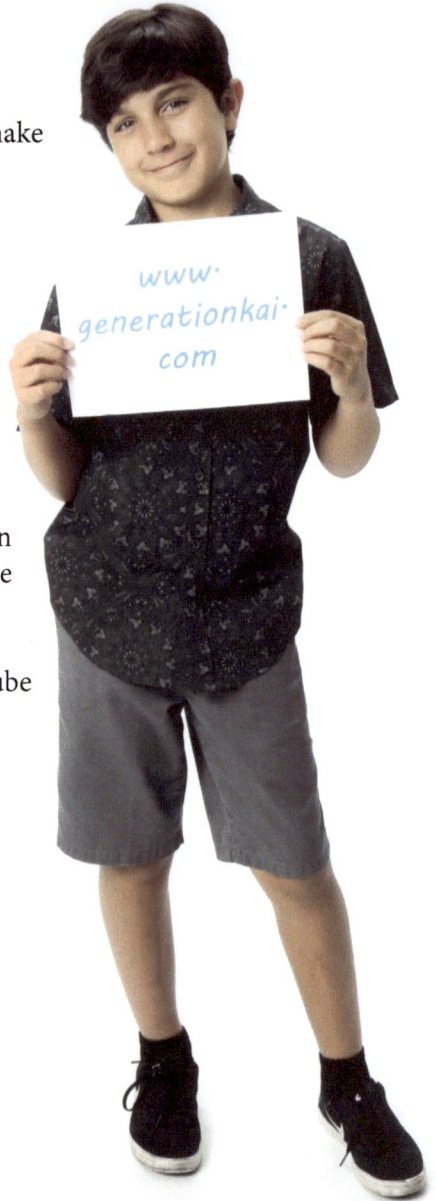

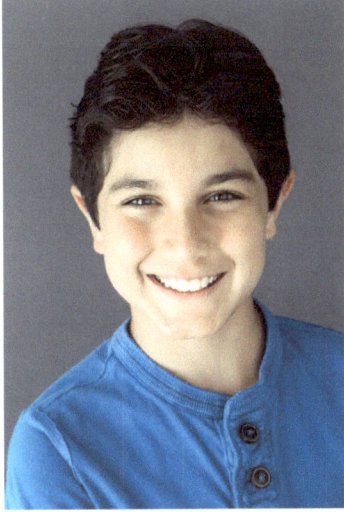

Kai Noah Anthony Nunziato-Cruz was born in 2006 and was 10 years old when he worked with his Moms on this book.

He loves eating and drinking healthy and loves staying active.

It's always been hard to keep up with him. :)

Aside from going to school, just a few of the ways he stays busy includes playing sports such as soccer, flag football and basketball.

He loves playing musical instruments such as the drums, piano and bells (xylophone).

He is extremely active in the theater world putting on shows at youth theaters in his area.

He loves to sing, dance and act.

He is also part of a performing group called Confetti.

He loves tumbling – (front and back flips) and he is excited to learn parkour - trying to move from one point to another in a complex environment by way of running, climbing, swinging, vaulting, jumping and rolling.

When he is not busy with all of that, he loves to read Big Nate and Diary of a Wimpy Kid books, play Legos (but mostly Lego guys), play Super Mario Brothers on his Wii and watch movies.

When it's not too hot in Phoenix he also loves playing outside with his sisters.

They love to ride bikes, skateboards, scooters and roller skates up and down their block.

He hopes this book helps you to learn more about your body and helps you to make better choices for yourself everyday.

He wants you to remember to **live on purpose, not on accident!**

And have fun being a happy and healthy kid!

Gastro Greens™

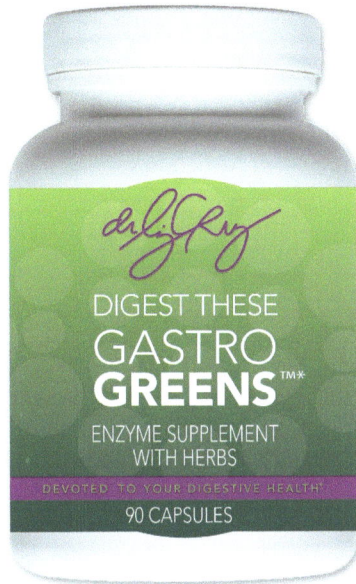

A variety of vitamins, minerals, and other essential nutrients are required to feed your body at the cellular level.

Lack of nutrition due to stressful lifestyle, poor eating habits, or food sensitivities can result in low energy, strength, and endurance.

This pure plant product with all natural phytonutrient complexes is not a "mega dose" of any one nutrient but rather a healthy balance of nutrients as found in nature.

Find out more at www.drlizcruz.com/products

Everyday Enzymes™

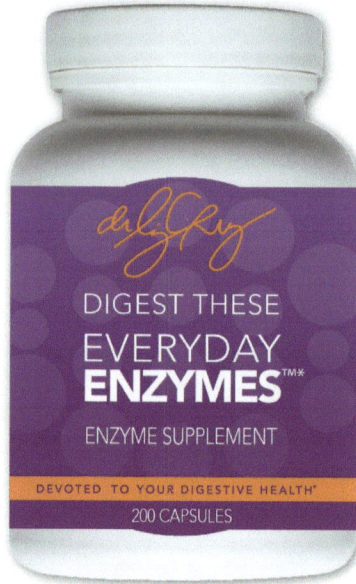

An enzyme supplement designed to assist the body in maximum digestion of nutrients, production of energy, and immune system support.

Supports the digestion of carbohydrates, proteins, and fats.

Excellent for those with a sensitive gut and experience GI discomfort.

Find out more at www.drlizcruz.com/products

Pleasant Probiotics™

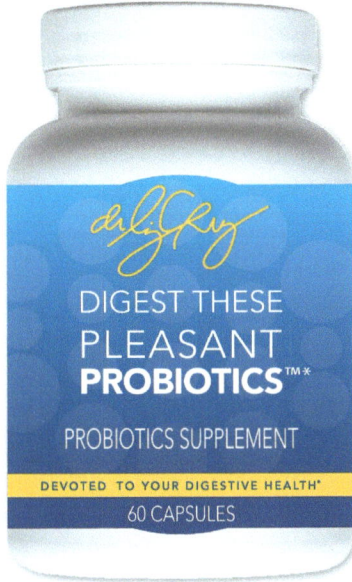

A comprehensive probiotic supplement designed to help promote gastrointestinal system health, assist with regularity, and support a healthy immune system.

This living bacteria also acts as a balancing agent for non-friendly bacteria located in the GI tract.

Find out more at www.drlizcruz.com/products

Delicate Detox™

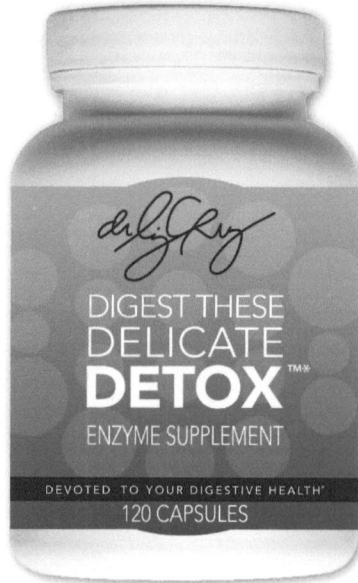

This is a gentle formula for those who are sensitive to detoxification.

This product will assist in maintaining optimal blood flow, immune function, and elimination of toxicity.

Find out more at www.drlizcruz.com/products

Super Salts™

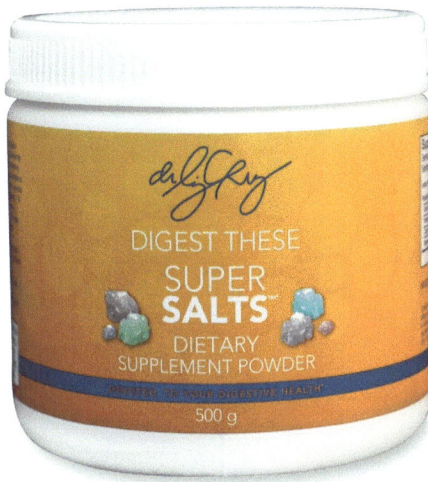

Super Salts™ is the "ultimate" antioxidant, anti-bacterial, anti-fungal, anti-inflammatory, anti-carcinogenic and anti-aging salts.

It contains the four key salts that are made up in the body allowing the body to replenish exactly what it is losing on a daily basis.

Specifically, they may aid in the reduction of dietary and metabolic acidity helping to maintain the alkaline design of the body.

Find out more at www.drlizcruz.com/products

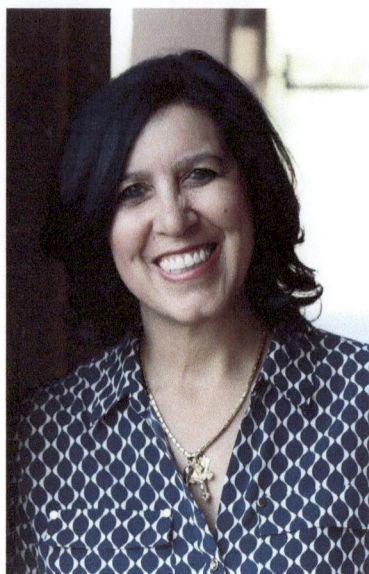

Dr. Cruz graduated from college in 1988 with a B.S. in Medical Technology.

Prior to Medical School, she taught English for one year in Bangkok Thailand.

In 1989, Dr. Cruz began her formal career in medicine by attending Loma Linda University School of Medicine in California.

During medical school, Dr. Cruz was part of a student / staff physician team, which provided relief work to the natives along the Amazon River.

She graduated from medical school in 1993 and then went on to do her Internal Medicine Internship under the auspices of the U.S. Navy at the Naval Hospital, Oakland, California.

Upon the closure of the Naval Hospital in Oakland, Dr. Cruz transferred and completed her internal medicine residency at the University of California, San Francisco.

In 1996, she was deployed to Guam to fulfill her commitment to the U.S. Navy.

While in Guam, she served as a Staff Internist at the U.S. Naval Hospital.

During her active duty years in the Navy, she received the Meritorious Unit Commendation Medal as well as the Humanitarian Service Medal and the National Defense Medal for service during Operation Desert Storm.

During her last two years in Guam, she was the Head of the Internal Medicine Division at the U.S. Naval Hospital.

In 2000, she went back to the University of California, San Francisco where she completed her training in Gastroenterology (GI).

In 2004, Dr. Cruz moved to Arizona to join the Arizona Medical Clinic in Peoria.

doing the full range of general gastroenterology including endoscopic procedures as well as hepatology.

In January 2007, she opened the doors to her own practice, Dr. Liz Cruz Partners in Digestive Health in Phoenix, Arizona.

In 2010, Dr. Cruz along with her life partner, Tina Nunziato began offering the Dr. Liz Cruz Wellness Program to educate patients on the very things that were causing their digestive issues.

After helping hundreds of patients improve and in some cases eliminate their digestive issues through detoxification, digestive restoration, nutrition, and proper hydration, Dr. Cruz decided to launch her products and services online.

Her "DNA for Digestive Health" 3 step program and the www. DigestiveRevolution.com online community she created are changing people's digestive health for good.

More information about her products and services can be found at www. drlizcruz.com and through her "Digest This™" podcast at www.digestthispodcast. com.

Dr. Cruz was born in Los Angeles, California and was raised in Orlando, Florida.

She speaks fluent Spanish and enjoys her family, traveling, jazz music, and photography.

Dr. Cruz is a Diplomate of the American Board of Internal Medicine and the American Board of Gastroenterology.

She is a member of the American College of Gastroenterology and the American Society for Gastrointestinal Endoscopy.

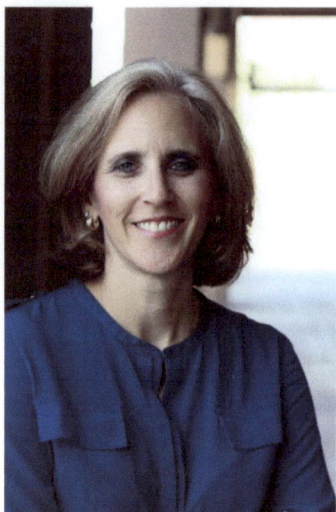

Tina Nunziato graduated from the Arizona State University College of Business Honors Program in 1996 with a Bachelor of Science in Marketing.

While attending ASU she was very active in the College of Business and the Residence Hall Association.

As the College of Business Honors Program Marketing Coordinator, Ms. Nunziato worked for four years creating programs for Honors students that still exist today.

As the President for the Residence Hall Association, Ms. Nunziato worked with other student organizations to better the life of all campus residents.

After graduation Ms. Nunziato took her first job out of college as a Marketing Analyst for a local telecommunications vendor, now Lucent Technologies.

She quickly moved out of market research and into business development as a Marketing Specialist where she worked on various new product and joint venture initiatives.

In addition, Ms. Nunziato was also responsible for managing projects produced by the students at Thunderbird Graduate School of Management.

In late 1999, during the dot-com boom, Ms. Nunziato moved to San Francisco to start a web-based software company with a fellow ASU College of Business graduate.

Focused on the park and recreation market, the company went through many strategy iterations before it found its niche.

In her role as COO and eventually CEO, Ms. Nunziato experienced all facets of business from raising capital and product design to selling, training and supporting customers.

In May of 2003, subsequent to selling her company to one of the industry competitors, Ms. Nunziato came back to her roots here in Arizona.

After rebuilding her network and consulting for various companies to determine her next step, she accepted a position with Carefx Corporation, a healthcare software company in Scottsdale.

As the Director of Marketing, Ms. Nunziato was responsible for all marketing initiatives including corporate and product messaging, sales tool development, managing strategic planning, and all print, web and tradeshow initiatives. Ms. Nunziato resigned from Carefx in 2006 to pursue Consult TNT with her father.

In 2007 Ms. Nunziato decided to try her hand in medicine when she started Dr. Liz Cruz Partners in Digestive Health with her life and business partner Dr. Elizabeth Cruz.

In addition to having a successful Gastroenterology practice Ms. Nunziato and Dr. Cruz took medicine one step further by offering a wellness program through their office.

In conjunction with and to support this business Ms. Nunziato went back to school to receive her Certificate in Holistic Nutrition in 2010.

Since then both businesses have been growing as they continue to heal patients year after year from digestive disease, sluggishness and weight gain.

In 2016 Ms. Nunziato was recognized by Arizona State University as a recipient of the Sun Devil 100.

The Sun Devil 100 Awards celebrate the achievements of Sun Devil-owned and Sun Devil-led businesses across the country.

www.ingramcontent.com/pod-product-compliance
Lightning Source LLC
Chambersburg PA
CBHW041226270326
41934CB00001B/17